Epilepsy in Telangana: A Complete Overview

Deepthi Shetty. M.Sc.

Faisal Ahmed Shariff, MSc.

Mohammed Aamir Niyaz, M.Sc.

Mohammad Shueb, M.Sc.

ISBN: 9798355336493
Imprint: Independently published

Front cover image by Deepthi Shetty.
Book design by Deepthi Shetty.

First printing edition 2022.

Table of Contents

Contents

CHAPTER 1: HISTORY OF TELANGANA

Telangana is the 29th and youngest state in the Indian Union. It became a political and legal state on June 2, 2014. It is also the 12th largest and the 12th most populated state in the country. However, it has a long history as an economic, social, cultural, and historical institution that goes back at least two thousand five hundred years or more.. (*Telangana State Portal History*, n.d.)

Nizams OF Hyderabad

Telangana was governed by the Satavahana Dynasty (230 BCE to 220 CE), the Kakatiya Dynasty (1083–1323), the Musunuri Nayaks (1326–1346), the Delhi Sultanate, the Bahmani Sultanate (1347–1512), the Golconda Sultanate (1512–1687), and the Asaf Jahi dynasty (1724–1950). The Mughal emperor, Aurangazeb, defeated the Qutub Shahi Kingdom at the Golconda Fort in 1687, taking control of the Deccan. After some time, Nizam-ul-Mulk defeated Mubariz Khan and seized Hyderabad in 1724. As the Nizams of

Hyderabad, their heirs controlled the empire state of Hyderabad. Qamar-ud-din Khan established the Asaf Jahi empire under the name Nizam-ul-Mulk and took control of the Deccan. Because of this, the Deccan kings were known as the Nizams. The difficult time in Telangana's history was the Mir Nizam Ali Khan period. Telangana, Northern Circars (or coastal Andhra), and Rayalaseemas were the three Telugu-speaking areas that make up the Nizam's domains. The Nizam was left with the Telangana Region, which later became known as Hyderabad's state. This means that the Telugu people were divided between the Madras presidency and Hyderabad state. And this went on for 150 years till India gained independence.

Gentleman's Agreement

Due to the violation of the gentlemen's agreement, the people of Telangana started a massive protest in 1969 and others demanded a separate state of Telangana. This movement is called the "Jai Telangana" movement. Students and government workers took the lead in this movement. The Telangana Praja Samiti (TPS), a new party, was established to represent Telangana's political demands. Nearly two decades later, the demand for Telangana became more popular due to the rise of K Chandrashekar Rao. He started his own political organization with the goal of creating a Telangana-specific state In the 2004 elections, he voted for Congress because it promised Telangana statehood(Seshan, 2018) but it didn't meet the demand that was expected. He then left the Congress Party to join the Telugu Desam Party. After KCR began a fast in 2009, the center was forced to give in to Telangana's demands because of the rising tension and KCR's failing health.

State Formation

On July 30, 2013, a proposal on the establishment of a separate Telangana state was passed by the Congress Working Committee. The bill passed many phases before being presented in the Indian Parliament in February 2014. Then KCR was appointed as Telangana's first chief minister, and it was eventually recognized as the 29th state. Until 2024, Hyderabad will remain as both the state and the capital(*The Telangana People's Movement: The Unfolding Political Culture on JSTOR*, n.d.).

Land, Language, Culture and Development

Telangana, often known as Telengana or Telingana, is a state in south-central India. It is bordered to the north by Maharashtra, to the northeast by Chhattisgarh and Odisha, to the southeast and south by Andhra Pradesh, and to the west by Karnataka. Telangana is mostly located in the Deccan uplands. It has a geographical area of 112,077 square kilometres.The hill region is around 1,600 feet (500 meters) high on average, with greater heights in the west and southwest and a sloping lower slope in the east and northeast where it meets the discontinuous line of the Eastern Ghats ranges. The valleys of the Godavari and Krishna rivers dominate irrigation in the north and south, respectively(*Telangana - History | Britannica*, n.d.).(*Telangana | Encyclopedia Article by TheFreeDictionary*, n.d.).

The Dravidian language, the state's official language and most popular dialect, is Telugu(*Language in India*, n.d.). Urdu is a language that is only spoken by a minority. Telugu is spoken by 77% of the state's citizens, Urdu by 12%, and other languages by 13%. The majority of the remaining communities converse in languages of the borderlands, such as Marathi,

Kannada, and Hindi. The state's scheduled tribes speak Lambadi (Banjari) and other languages(*Telangana Dialect - Wikipedia*, n.d.)(Telangana Dialect-Wikipedia, n.d.). Telugu became the official language of the government after Hyderabad State joined the new Republic of India in 1948.

Hyderabad and Warangal, the cultural centers of Telangana, are well known for their wealth and illustrious historical buildings, including the Charminar, Qutb Shahi Tombs, Warangal Fort, Paigh Tombs, Falaknuma Palace, Chowmahalla Palace, Kakatiya Kala Thoranam, Thousand Pillar Temple, and the Bhongir Fort in Yadadri Bhuvanagiri district(<i>Telangana | Encyclopedia Article by TheFreeDictionary</i>, n.d.). Some of the most well-known diamonds in the world were created in the Golconda region. The colorless Orlov (Russia), the Nizam, and the Jacob (India). Folk arts such as Kolatam, Perini Shivatandavam, Gusadi Dance, and Burra Katha, as well as folk songs, classical music, and painting, have a long history in the state (*Huge Challenges Ahead for New Telangana Tourism Corporation | Hyderabad News - Times of India*, n.d.).

The many art forms produced by Telangana's various tribes and areas, including paintings, handicrafts made of wood and metal, and textiles, reflect the artistic character of the locals.

Hyderabad is home to a large number of museums, temples, and other buildings of cultural significance. Furthermore, the historical sites in and around Hyderabad and Warangal are well-known for documenting the centuries-long Muslim rule in the region.

Most of think us that Telangana is only famous for Hyderabadi Biriyanis, as there are many types of biriyanis prepared in these region but besides biriyani there are many other food items from these region which we are not aware. Malidalu, Sarva Pindi, Garijalu, Golichina Mamsam, Sakinalu, Pachi pulusu, Chegodilu, Qubani ka Meetha, Thunti Koora, Bachali Kura are some of the famous foods in Telangana. Also it is famous for Karachi Biscuits.

Telangana is expanding more quickly than the national average and the majority of the states in India. Telangana's nominal GDP is up 21.8% from pre-pandemic levels in 2021–2022, whereas India's nominal GDP has only grown by 17.8% during the same period. The COVID-19 pandemic had an impact on Telangana's economy, but despite this, the state was able to raise its GSDP at current prices in 2020–21 compared to the previous year. The GSDP of Telangana State in the financial year 2013–14, when it was formed, was Rs 5,05,849 crore. By the fiscal year 2021-2022, it had risen to Rs 11,54,860 crore.Hyderabad is also the fifth-largest contributor to India's overall GDP(*GSDP: Telangana's GSDP More than Doubles to Rs 11.55 Lakh Cr in 8 Yrs - The Economic Times*, n.d.).

Although the pandemic had a severe impact on the industries and services sectors in India, those sectors had a significant recovery in the years 2021–2022; their respective values rose from -1.63% and -4.65% in 2020–2021 to 25.93% and 17.57% in 2021–2022, respectively. Agriculture, particularly the cultivation of rice, has traditionally dominated the economy of Telangana. Agriculture and related industries saw a significant increase in current price GVA of 12.24% and 9.09% in 2020–2021 and 2021–2022, respectively (*Telangana | History, Map, Population, Capital, & Government | Britannica*, n.d.).

The majority of the state government's expenditures come from revenue and capital revenues. The state government had planned revenue receipts of Rs. 1,76,127 crore and capital revenues of Rs. 45,560 crore for the financial year 2021–22 BE (Budget Estimates). In comparison to India GS's average of 57.7%, the state's own revenue during 2017 to 2020 amounted to 73.8% of total revenue collections. Taxes are collected by the Commercial Taxes Department of the Government of Telangana, which shows the state's significant growth in revenue. They nearly doubled, rising from Rs. 27,700 crore in 2014-15 to Rs. 52,436 crore in 2020-21.

Telangana state is improving the state economy and generating a lot of job opportunities for its people by giving more importance to the industrial sector. The industrial sector's GVA increased by 20.23% in Telangana in 2021–2022. At the national level, the industrial sector's GVA increased by 25.93% in nominal terms during the same span of time. By covering stamp duty, electricity costs, granting interest and investment subsidies, financial assistance, and other help with quality control and patent registration, the state provides incentives to entrepreneurs under

Telangana State Industrial Development and Entrepreneur Advancement (T-IDEA) for establishing industries.

Telangana is listed in the top 10 for affordable talent in the global ecosystem, the top 15 for "bang for the buck" in the global ecosystem, and the top 5 for funding in the Asian ecosystem. There are more than 6,500 registered startups in the Telangana ecosystem, including four unicorns and a number of companies developing goods and services for a worldwide market(*Telangana among Top-10 Global Startup Ecosystems*, n.d.).

Telangana is one of the fastest growing states in India. Seven Telangana villages were awarded the Sansad Adarsh Gramina Yojana and the state also received a national award by the Ministry of Rural Development, Government of India for 19 Telangana Villages.

Telangana State has provided the country and the globe with an innovative development model. It has improved, functioning as an example to the rest of India.

CHAPTER 2: HEALTH CARE SYSTEM IN TELANGANA

In health care system Telangana is affordable and standard than many other cities in India. The state main is to improve health care services and provide prestigious treatment.

Being a new state the government is slowly building on its health schemes and infrastructure. Telangana has become the one of the best performing state in the health care sector. And it is considered to be top performer when it comes to health care.

Health care system is mainly focuses on socio-economic factors like education, income, economy, standard of living, housing, sanitation, employment, standard of living, water supply and health care awareness etc.

Telangana has consistently done well in the performance of health of a population. In last few years, Telangana's health care parameters like maternal and infant mortality rates , under 5-mortality and total fatality rates have outperformed the national averages(*Telangana to Spend Rs*

10,000 Crore on Improving Public Healthcare | Deccan Herald, n.d.).

After the formation of Telangana, the government has allocated and spent a Rs. 677.42 crore only towards procurement of new diagnostic medical equipment, infrastructure and financial support for different schemes and now it has allocated Rs.1000 crore to set up government medical colleges in all districts of the state in next two years.

The state has improved the quality of medical equation and it concerned about medical states and launched a new medical colleges in the state. The authorities also set aside nearly Rs.300 crore to build a new medical college and have total 10 government medical colleges. During Covid-19 pandemic, when there was no specific infrastructure available to treat covid patients, the health department played a very well role in creating special oxygen lines, ICU beds and Covid Care facilities and giving training to health workers.

Reliance on the private healthcare system is the highest in Telangana compared to other states in the country. As per the NSSO data on health survey around 78 percent of all hospitalisations in a year takes place in private hospitals.

Telangana came up with many initiatives. Here are the some of the state government providing health care facilities to the state:

Arogya siri Scheme

It is the scheme of all the health initiatives of the state government to provide quality healthcare to the poor. Its main aim is to improve the quality of medical care for the treatment of diseases involving like surgeries, hospitalization and therapies to the access of BPL families. Through this scheme, the government will distribute free health and hygiene kits to the girl students in grade 7 to 12 in all the government schools and junior colleges. also for heart, liver, and bone marrow transplantation government assistance upto Rs 2lakhs to Rs 5 lakhs.

KCR kit Scheme

It was launched in the year 2017. Its main aim is to significantly reduce the toll of maternal and pregnancy wastage. Also it was adopted to ensure safe pregnancy and newborn survival. This scheme provide the expectant mothers to receive financial assistance of

Rs.13,000 for a girl child and Rs.12,000 for a male child. This kit is specially for the new parents who doesn't have ability to purchase item themselves with 16 essential health and nutrition items.

Midwifery initiative

It is launched to provide autonomy to pregnant women in making their own choice of birthing, reduction of C-sections by encouraging natural birthing and promotes respectful maternity care.

Amma vodi Scheme

This scheme provides the transportation to all pregnant woman to ANC checkups to delivery and postnatal care. Around 300 ambulances under this scheme with pick-up and drop back services to the mother and child.

Kanti Velugu

This programme is about "Avoidable Blindness free Telangana" launched in the year 2018. This scheme conducts eye screening and vision test for the citizens of the state and giving free spectacles to the people.

Arogya Lakshmi Scheme

This scheme mainly takes care of pregnant and lactating women as well as infants by giving the complete nutrition to them.

Electronic Intensive Care Unit(eICU)

This scheme services in the remote areas by providing critical care services. Each having 10 beds with 15 peripheral ICUs.

ST- Elavation Myocardial Infarction

This is mainly for Heart case. The public health facilities are now equipped with STEMI and spoke model. 82000 ECGs have been transmitted and in 3446 critical cases of which 1626 cases are STEMI cases.

Basti Dawakhanas

This was launched in the year 2018 by greater Hyderabad Muncipal Corporation in Telangana. The main goal of this programme is to strengthening the primary health care in the state. It offers free medicines and consultation and also a variety of diagnostic tests. This has doctors, Asha workers and nurses.

CHAPTER 3: EPILEPSY IN TELANGANA

One of the most prevalent and severe neurologic disorders, epilepsy, is still poorly understood in terms of its detailed pathophysiology and, thus, the reason for most of its treatments. Epilepsy is a common neurological disorder that affects 1 in 100 people. Moreover, 10% of children will experience at least one seizure during their lifetime. There will be many questions after someone is diagnosed with epilepsy because they need to know what to do and what not to do, how to manage the condition, and what will happen to them in terms of their profession and marriage. (Stafstrom & Carmant, 2015).Epilepsy is a group of disorders that reflect underlying brain malfunctions and can have a number of origins. It is not a single disease entity. With a frequency of about 50 new cases each year per 100,000 people, As a result of the developing brain's greater sensitivity to seizures, around 75% of cases of epilepsy start in childhood (Buckley & Holmes, 2016). In the 1960s, epilepsy and stroke were the only neuroepidemiological conditions that were studied in

India. Worldwide, 50 million people have epilepsy, with the majority living in developing nations. There are around 10 million epileptics in India. Stigma, exclusion, limitations, overprotection, and isolation may be experienced by patients with epilepsy. For the patient and their families, seizures and the possibility of recurrent seizures can have psychological effects.

In Telangana, Four lakh people are suffering from epilepsy, with a prevalence rate of one percent of the population, however urban areas have a higher frequency than rural ones. Many members of the family are not even aware that there is such a thing as epilepsy disorder or that it can be controlled or treated. It is crucial to spread awareness of the fact that treatments are very cost-effective. In rural areas, 90 percent of patients avoid therapy, compared to 75 percent of patients who choose to receive it. These patients don't get to the healthcare facilities because of different cultural beliefs, poverty, and insufficient facilities for health delivery

As the world's population ages, neurological disorders become more common, making it difficult for health-care systems to remain effective, particularly in low-

and middle-income countries.There were many different types of neurological conditions found, including common conditions like epilepsy, febrile convulsions, headache, cerebro-vascular disorders, stroke, tremors, and mental retardation. People aged 35 to 45 who experience mental disorders suffer most commonly from depression and anxiety disorders. Epilepsy (36%), headache (17%), stroke (16%), and diseases of the peripheral nervous system (13.2%) are the most common neurological disorders. According to the survey, only 19% of respondents in Hyderabad knew about at least one symptom, while 81% were unaware of the word "brain stroke" and 78% were familiar with the term "brain stroke."

Anxiety disorders made up 19%, while cases of depression made up 33.8% in Telangana. The period of mental health treatment is lengthy, and it includes regular medical visits, medication, and frequent prescription changes. The increasing burdens of high blood pressure, increased sugar, air pollution, obesity, and dietary dangers are blamed for the growth in neurological disorders. Stroke is the leading cause of death, with an incidence rate of 37.9%. Stroke-related disabilities increase the socioeconomic stress on families. Men experience migraines at a rate of 19%, and the headache incidence is 17.9%. 10.5% of those with epilepsy have cerebral palsy, while 5.7% of women and 5.9% of men have epilepsy (*Burden of Neurological Disorders Have Doubled in 30 Years in India*, n.d.).

The disease burden of epilepsy is significant in the state when compared to the incidence of epilepsy detection in children. In the past three years, the state has seen an average of 12,000 new cases of epilepsy per year. Childhood epilepsy is becoming more common. It is increasingly being discovered as a result of new studies and technological developments. In its neurology, general medicine, and paediatric outpatient clinics, a regional large tertiary care teaching hospital that serves the region enrolled 160 patients with recent onset seizures between 2011 and 2014. Brain imaging was carried out in each of the mentioned patients. Using a commercial immunoglobulin G-ELISA test, neurocysticercosis (NCC) was diagnosed antigenically. Whether or not radio imaging confirms the diagnosis (Pappala et al., 2016).People turn to spiritual leaders instead of medical personnel for help with neurological disorders because they feel embarrassed by them. However, epilepsy is not commonly recognised.

Case Study 1

The Mamata Medical College and General Hospital conducted a neurological disorder study in the Khammam district of Telangana state for 3 years. After receiving written consent, the patients who were willing to participate in the study and were visiting the neurology department were included. All of the patients were divided into groups based on their problems, and a history of risk factors was maintained. Percentages were used to express every value. This study had 1326 patients in total. All of them ranged in age from 35 to 75, and 672 of them were men and 654 were women. Epilepsy was the most common neurological condition in this study; 482 out of the total patients (36.3%) had it. Headaches (228 patients) and strokes (221 patients) were the next most common neurological disorders. Out of 221 stroke patients, 48 passed away over a three-year period, 128 survived with long-term injuries and impairments, and the majority of survivors suffered from severe depression. With a ratio of 1:9:1, neurological problems were more prevalent in the rural population than in the urban population(K, 2017)

Case Study 2

During the period of a year, from February 2017 to January 2018, the department of pediatrics at Maheshwara Medical College and Hospital in Patancheru, Telangana, conducted a study on the occurrence and clinical spectrum of seizures among children. There were 75 cases in total that were admitted to the paediatric unit with complaints of seizures. The inclusion criteria and exclusion criteria were both present. The age range for the inclusion criterion was 1 week to 14 years, with both genders represented. Among the exclusion criteria is age, more than 14 years. Patient demographics such as age and gender, seizure type, accompanying symptoms, family history of seizure or epilepsy, birth history, developmental history, past history of seizures, and treatment history were collected. 960 patients in total were hospitalized in the paediatric unit over the period of a year, and 75 of those cases had both acute and unprovoked seizures and newborn seizures.

Unprovoked seizure patients had to receive regular care and treatment (Sastry & Reddy, 2018). According to statistics, 1 in 100 people tend to develop this disorder, which is most common in elderly people and children.

Case Study 3

Another study was carried out in the Indian state of Telangana's Moinabad mandal of Ranga Reddy District. The WHO Basis study shows a significant urban-rural divide in cardiovascular risk factor knowledge and medication use for stroke prevention, with less than 25% of rural participants using prescribed medicine. The recommended study would identify the stroke risk factors in the rural Telangana population and give health care professionals a guide for implementing treatment and control measures. Between July 2016 and December 2017, the population of Moinabad Mandal in Telangana, India's Ranga Reddy District, was investigated. There are over 13,000 families in 26 villages, making up the approximately 56,000 people that live in Moinabad mandal. About 27,000 women and 29,000 men make up the population. Among all people, 75% belong to the general caste, 25% to the scheduled caste, and none to the scheduled tribes. Through a door-to-door survey, the patients were selected by line listing from the village of Moinabad. The characteristics were hospital visits, current medical treatment, medical reports, computed tomography scans or magnetic resonance imaging reports where available, demographic information including age, gender, and educational level, history of stroke (previous or family), and medical data. A physical examination includes checking blood pressure (BP), collecting blood samples for lipid profile analysis. As a result, in Moinabad Mandal, the estimated crude prevalence of stroke is 257 per 100,000 people. Stroke prevalence among men is 344 per 100,000, but it is only 163 per 100,000 among women. Given the high rate of strokes in rural Telangana, the state faces a serious public health issue.

Case Study 4

The medical outpatient department at Osmania General Hospital studied 50 cases of newly diagnosed focal seizures that were admitted to the hospital's medical wards between January 2013 and June 2014. In terms of the nature of the condition, the form of the illness and its effects on people and families, epilepsy is a major public health issue. In this study, the clinical characteristics and etiology of newly developing focal seizures in people older than 18 years old will be examined. Depending on the etiological factors, all patients were started on the proper antiepileptic medications and other medications. Neurocysticercosis patients responded well to albendazole, steroids, and anti-epileptic medicines worked well for treating Neurocysticercosis patients.(Journal, n.d.)

Case Study 5

The occurrence of psychiatric problems among Hyderabad's epilepsy patients is the reason for this study. At the Malla Reddy Institute of Medical Sciences in Hyderabad, 100 patients who had been diagnosed with epilepsy according to the ILAE 2014 criteria had their respective data analyzed. This contains both inclusion and exclusion criteria, with the inclusion criterion that the patient has been diagnosed with epilepsy according to ILAE criteria and has been using anti-epileptic drugs (AED) for more than six months with informed consent. When exclusion criteria Patients who are older than 60 and wasn't taking an AED, however, may have neurological deficits or mental impairment. The principal investigator gave a survey to the patient with his or her permission in Telugu, Hindi, or English using the well-established Washington Psychological Seizure Inventory (WPSI) scale. The patients were examined by asking a total of 24 questions over 7 domains. Finally, 100 patients who passed the inclusion and exclusion criteria were finally included in the trial with the range of ages between 15 to 57. The ratio of men to women was 7:3. All of the patients were from Hyderabad's suburbs. Only 19% of people have reported having depression symptoms and difficulty coping with many areas of daily life under the emotional component category. However, the majority of them experienced anxiety, embarrassment (70%), tension (62%), and emotional upset (62%). 30% of people with epilepsy felt dissatisfied about their condition and had low self-esteem, but the majority (70%) were embarrassed by upcoming seizures.

Epilepsy adversely affects psychosocial functioning in a variety of ways that affect physical, psychological, social, occupational, and economic aspects of life.(*Aim & Scope - (IAIM)*, n.d.)

Public Awareness

A comprehensive epilepsy program has been launched by Hyderabad-based Star Hospitals for the benefit of thousands of patients in the region. According to hospital sources, the primary goal of this program is to give patients the best treatment planning possible using a variety of therapeutic methods. (*Star Hospitals Launches Comprehensive Epilepsy Programme in Hyderabad*, n.d.).

The Epilepsy Foundation has taken out public campaigns. EASE, an Epilepsy Awareness and Social Empowerment Society (Non-Profit) have conducted various awareness campaigns about epilepsy in Hyderabad. The goal is to ensure that people with epilepsy may participate in all aspects of Indian society. This main aim is to eliminate misunderstandings and prohibitions about this disease, especially in rural areas, by providing information and education. On International Epilepsy Day, they also worked along with Nizam College in Hyderabad, and institutions' students and faculty took part in a walk to raise awareness about epilepsy.

Also, the epilepsy awareness was conducted at Prathima Hospital Kaachiguda, Hyderabad to increase awareness among people about epilepsy. People can learn about epilepsy through a variety of sources, including their friends and family, the news and entertainment media, the Internet, and social media.

CHAPTER 4: EPILEPSY AND NEUROLOGICAL DOCTORS OF TELANGANA

The government should aim towards improving the services for issues related to neurological conditions as there are no adequate neurologists. There is only one neurologist for every 5 lakh people in our nation, which only adds up to 2500. The ideal ratio, according to WHO, is 1 doctor for every 1 lakh people. Hence, the number of neurologists in the country should be increased so as to maintain the ratio as per WHO(*'Shortage of Neurologists in Country'* - *The Hindu*, n.d.).

There are only 350 million neurologists across the world. The Telangana population is around 3.5 million, out of which half of the population are the residents of Hyderabad. These patients' neurological conditions and medical care are undisclosed. According to renowned neurologists in Hyderabad, a small number of epilepsy types need permanent treatment for the majority of patients in order to manage or prevent seizures. (*Experts Say Telangana Needs More Neurologists- The New Indian Express*, n.d.).

Some of the best epilepsy specialist doctors in Telangana state are listed below.

Sita Jayalakshmi, M.D.

Dr. Sita Jayalakshmi is a best consultant neurologist at KIMS in Hyderabad, India. She had a prestigious career as a neurologist and carries with her a high level of knowledge and thoroughness in patient care. She worked in a variety of positions at prestigious healthcare facilities. She has almost 20 years of experience as a neurologist with epilepsy and epilepsy surgery and served as an associate professor of neurology at Nizam's Institute of Medical Sciences. At KIMS, Dr. Sita leads a program for epilepsy surgery care. Their team has completed more than 750 such operations(*Best Neurology Hospital in Hyderabad | Top Neurology in Hyderabad*, n.d.)The American Academy of Neurology, the Indian Epilepsy Association, the Indian Epilepsy Society, the Indian Academy of Neurology, and the Neurological Society of India are just a few of the national and international associations she belongs to. She is on the International Journal of Epilepsy editorial board and examines publications related to epilepsy. In national and international journals including Epilepsy Research, Epilepsy & Behavior, Seizure, Clinical Neurology and Neurosurgery, Acta Neurologica Scandanavica, Neurology India, Annals of the Indian Academy of Neurology, and many others, Dr. Sita has published more than 90 articles. She has written chapters for neuroscience textbooks(*Neuro Specialist Hyderabad | Best Neurologist In Hyderabad*, n.d.).

Dr. Habib G. Pathan

With more than 18 years of experience in paediatric neurology, Dr. Habib G. Pathan is the top paediatric neurologist in Hyderabad. He treats all types of neurological disorders, syndromes, and defects in children, including developmental delays, learning and selective attention difficulties such as ADHD (attention deficit hyperactivity disorder), Angelman syndrome, movement disorders like dystonia, dystonia, dyskinesia, myopathies, and muscular dystrophies, as well as headaches, migraines, epilepsy, febrile seizures, strokes, and muscle disorders like hypotonia, dystonia, dystonia, dyskines. As a fellowship-trained child neurologist, Dr. Khan carefully manages a variety of neurological diseases, including the most difficult and complex ones. He manages all neurological problems that affect children. He is Hyderabad's most in-demand child neurologist due to his extensive experience, skill, and expertise in diagnosing and treating all types of neurological disorders in children(*Best Pediatric Neurologist in Hyderabad | Dr Habib Pathan |*, n.d.).

Dr. Neehar Potluri:

Dr. Neehar Potluri has 22 years of experience as a general physician and neurologist in Kukatpally, Hyderabad. He treats patients at Neehar Neuro Center and OMNI hospitals. He received his MBBS from the Institute of Medical Sciences, Banaras Hindu University (IMS-BHU) in 2000, his MD in general medicine from the same institution in 2003, and his DM in neurology from the KJMC in Lucknow in 2005. He belongs to the Indian Medical Association and the Indian Academy of Neurology (IMA). Nerve and muscle disorders, brain mapping, intra-arterial thrombolysis, brain aneurysm surgery, and intravenous therapy are just a few of the services the doctor provides(*Dr. Neehar Potluri - Neurologist - Book Appointment Online, View Fees, Feedbacks | Practo*, n.d.)

Dr. K. Krishna Reddy

In Hyderabad, Dr. K. Krishna Reddy is an experienced neurosurgeon and neurologist. He has 35 years of experience in the medical industry. He received the IAM Award for his contributions to the medical field. He received his MBBS from Osmania University in 1966, his DM in neurology from Osmania University in 1984, and his MD in general medicine from Osmania University in 1972. He currently provides consultations at Yashoda Hospitals Malakpet in Malakpet (Hyderabad). He is a respected IAM member(*Dr. K. Krishna Reddy - Neurosurgeon in Hyderabad | ClinicSpots*, n.d.).

.Some of the conditions neurologist Dr. K Krishna Reddy treats are: Epilepsy, Neurosyphilis, Meningitis, Encephalitis, Brachial Plexus,Rupture, Brain Cancer, Myelitis, Brachial Plexus, and Brain Stroke.

Dr. Komal Kumar RN,

Dr. Komal Kumar, RN, has more than 26 years of experience. He's held a position at Yashoda Hospitals. He is consulting at Janapareddy Hospital right now. He has vast knowledge about neurology, epilepsy, neurological disorders, stroke disorders, cervical spine decompression, status epilepticus, and neuro infections(*Dr. R. N. Komal Kumar,Neurologist in Secunderabad,Hyderabad Reviews,Contact Number,Fees | 365Doctor*, n.d.). The Neurological Society of India recognizes Dr. Komal Kumar, RN, as a member. Dr. Komal Kumar RN received his MBBS degree from the Dr. NTR University of Health Sciences in Andhra Pradesh. Dr. Komal Kumar RN then continued on to get a DM in neurology from the Dr. NTR University of Health Sciences in Andhra Pradesh.

Dr. Suma Kandukuri,

Dr. Suma K, She is a consultant neurophysician at Suma Neuro Care, Chanda Nagar. She received an MD in pediatrics from Niloufer Hospital and a DM in neurology from Osmania Medical College (Osmania Medical College). She has been devotedly treating patients from the Neurology department for more than five years, successfully diagnosing and curing their ailments. She is well trained in managing critical neurological cases like spinal cord disorders, refractory seizures, GBS, encephalopathies, meningitis, etc. knowledgeable about the diagnosis and treatment of a variety of degenerative diseases, including epilepsy and fits treatment, dementia, Parkinson's disease, and other movement disorders(*Dr. Suma K. - Neurologist - Book Appointment Online, View Fees, Feedbacks | Practo*, n.d.).

Dr.Sujit Kumar Vidiyala

In Secunderabad, Hyderabad, Dr. Sujit Kumar Vidiyala conducts neurosurgery and orthopedic spine surgery. He has 22 years of experience in these domains. At the Krishna Institute of Medical Sciences in Secunderabad, Hyderabad, Dr. Sujit Kumar Vidiyala does have a practice. In 1993, he received his MBBS at J.S.S. Medical College in Mysore, and in 1997, he earned his MCh in neurosurgery at the Nizam Institute of Medical Sciences in Hyderabad. He belongs to the AP and Telangana Neurological Societies, the Neurological Society of India, and the Society for Skull

Base Surgery of India (SBSSI). The doctor provides a variety of procedures, including peripheral neurosurgery, brain tumor surgery, vagus nerve stimulation for epilepsy, and cerebrovascular surgery(*Dr. Sujit Kumar Vidiyala - Neurosurgeon - Book Appointment Online, View Fees, Feedbacks | Practo*, n.d.).

Dr. Pranathi Gutta

With over 20 years of experience, Dr. Pranathi Gutta is a recognized paediatric neurologist. She is knowledgeable about neurological problems, including treatment of cerebral palsy, canalith repositioning (CR), vagus nerve stimulation for epilepsy, and video EEG.

In 2001, she graduated from Osmania Medical College in Hyderabad with an MBBS. Her membership in the Royal College of Paediatrics and Child Health was later earned in 2005. (MRCPCH, London, Glasgow, or Edinburgh). She has strong connections with esteemed institutions.

Numerous honors and recognitions have been awarded to her(*Dr Pranathi Gutta | Paediatric Neurologist in Hyderabad - Apollo Health City Jubilee Hills*, n.d.).

Dr. Sandhya Manorenj

After receiving an MBBS from Trivandrum Medical College in 1998, the specifications for a 9-month residency in general medicine there. In 2001, I participated in a three-year DNB (Diplomate of National Board) general medicine residency course at Choithram Hospital and Research Institute in Indore. I received a DNB in General Medicine degree in 2004 from the National Board of Examination. In 2004, he won the Dr. Sam G.P. Moses gold medal for general medicine in 2004 for ranking first nationally. I completed a super specialized post doctoral degree in neurology at the Apollo Institute of Medical Science and Health City, which is Joint Commission International (JCI) organ specific approved for stroke. The National Board of Examination awarded the Diplomate in National Board (DNB) in Neurology degree in 2009(*Dr. Sandhya Manorenj - Neurologist -

Book Appointment Online, View Fees, Feedbacks | Practo, n.d.).

Dr. M. Chandra Sekhar Reddy

Dr. M. Chandra Sekhar Reddy works at his own highly specialized hospital called MCS Neuro Hospital at KPHB, Hyderabad. Additionally, he has 18 years of experience in neurology. He formerly worked as a Chief Consultant Neuro Physician at several corporate hospitals, including Medicity, Global Hospitals, NIMS, and Narayana Hrudayala. He contributes to a number of professional associations, including the American Academy of Neurology, the World Federation of Neurology, the European Federation of Neurological Societies, and the Indian Academy of Neurology. Dr. M.Chandra Sekhar Reddy is currently providing services and treatments like Electromyography (EMG), Neurological Problems, Movement Disorders, Epilepsy Treatment, Nerve & Muscle Disorders, and many more(*Dr. M.Chandra Sekhar Reddy, Neurologist - Kukatpally, Hyderabad. | Drlogy*, n.d.).

Dr. Amitava Ray

He is a Paediatric Neurologist at Apollo Hospital, Secunderbad , Hyderabad. He has 22 years of experience in neurology. He mainly specializes in spine surgery , brain tumor surgery, headaches/migraine, and neurological issues such as epilepsy, Parkinson's diseases etc. He did his MBBS degree from the Medical College, Calcutta in 1992 and his FRCS-General Surgery from the Royal College of Surgeons of Edinburgh, UK in 1997. He has over 50 research articles on neurology. He is also a member of the Indian Society of Paediatric Neurosurgery and the Society of British Neurological Surgeons(*Dr Amitava Ray | Neurosurgeon in Hyderabad - Apollo Health City Jubilee Hills*, n.d.).

Dr. Suresh Babu P.

He is a senior consultant and neurologist at AIG hospital in Telangana. He holds an MBBS and a DM in neurology from Christian Medical College, Vellor. He specialized in treating epilepsy, seizures, strokes, dementia, chronic headaches, etc. (*Dr. Suresh Babu*

Consultant Neurologist & Epileptologist in Hyderabad, n.d.).

Subhash Kaul, M.D.

He is the best neurologist in Hyderabad. He is a senior consultant neurologist and associate professor at KIMS hospital. He holds his MBBS and MD from the Government Medical College, Srinagar. He has a special interest in stroke therapies. He also treats back and neck pain, paralysis, hemorrhage, head infection treatment, etc. (*Dr. Subhash Kaul | Best Neuro Surgeon in Hyderabad | Alzheimers Specialist in Hyderabad,* n.d.).

A neurologists helps in healing problems like epilepsy, strokes, etc. If the pain is not decreased by the medication, then one should visit a neurosurgeon for a surgical option.

CHAPTER 5: NEUROLOGY HOSPITALS IN TELANGANA

Eliminating side effects is the aim of epilepsy treatment delivered in a specialized epilepsy hospital. additionally, providing complete therapeutic and diagnostic assistance to those suffering from uncontrolled seizures.Board-certified neurosurgeons in Hyderabad with vast experience provide complete treatment options for both adults and children using the newest state of technology.There are numerous hospitals in Telangana that treat epilepsy that are listed below with details:

KIMS Hospital

With facilities throughout Telangana, Andhra Pradesh, and Maharashtra, The Krishna Institute of Medical Sciences (KIMS)Hospitals is one of the major corporate healthcare companies in India. It offers multidisciplinary integrated healthcare services. It was founded by Dr. Bhaskar Rao Bollineni in 2000.The

KIMS Group's headquarters are located in KIMS Secunderabad. Patients not only travel to the department of neurology from all over the states of Telangana and Andhra Pradesh, but also from other parts of India and abroad, making it a center of excellence and tertiary care referral hospital. Clinical treatment and research efforts in a variety of post are actively pursued by the department.Since its establishment in 2004, the Department of Neurology at KIMS Hospitals has placed the needs of its patients first, making it one of the top neurology hospitals in Hyderabad and India.

An experienced group of Specialists who have performed more than 650 epilepsy surgeries provide epilepsy surgery care at KIMS. The team is made up of the neurosurgeon Dr. Manas Panigrahi, the pahologist Dr. Sailaja M, the nuclear medicine experts Drs. Pushpalatha Sudhakar and Praveen Kumar, the radiologist Dr. VSV Rammohan, and the clinical psychologist Dr. Shanmukhi.(*Best Hospital For Epilepsy Treatment Surgery in Hyderabad*, n.d.)

Senior Consultant Neurologist Dr. Sita Jayalakshmi is particularly interested in pre - surgical examination to identify the seizure site. Modern facilities are available at KIMS for both surgery and pre-surgical examination of patients with epilepsy. Three devices for long-term continuous VEEG monitoring were established in the VEEG lab.

During the evaluation of patients for epilepsy surgery, Dr. Pushpalatha Sudhakar and Dr. Praveen Kumar Singa, Consultants at the Nuclear Medicine Department, use ictal SPECT and PET Scans to identify the abnormal area. Technology utilized in epilepsy center includes EEG, Neuroimaging, Brain mapping, and electronic assistive technology(*Kims Hospitals*, n.d.-a). Epileptic surgery is one of the epilepsy treatments that KIMS focuses in. The most experienced epilepsy specialists who have dealt with various cases and are familiar with how each case functions with various patients provide these procedures or treatments.(*Kims Hospitals*, n.d.-b)

A major achievement, for the Krishna Institute of Medical Sciences (KIMS) Hospitals, is that it has performed 1,000 epilepsy surgeries.When medication failed to control a child's or an adult's seizures, epilepsy surgery was performed. Surgery is used to remove a part of the brain where seizures frequently occur when anti-seizure drugs, which are the first line of treatment, are not able to control seizures in patients.

The Epilepsy Monitoring Laboratory records and studies the electroencephalograms (EEGs) of patient candidates, which helps in classifying the type and locations of the observed seizures. Furthermore, a combination of modern brain imaging tests such as 3TMRI scans, PET scans, and SPECT scans may be used(Gourie-Devi, 2014)

Another case is, A 32-year-old patient has undergone Deep Brain Stimulation (DBS) therapy to help with the symptoms of Parkinson's disease at Krishna Institute of Medical Sciences (KIMS) Hospitals in Secunderabad after being diagnosed with a rare ailment with symptoms of tightness in the hands and legs and trouble walking, similar to Parkinson's disease.The first automated Deep Brain Stimulation (DBS) procedure was performed at KIMS Hospital(*Hyderabad Doctors Give New Lease of Life to 3-Year-Old Epileptic Child*, n.d.).

Epilepsy surgery using a robotic system with artificial intelligence is available at KIMS Hospital, along with brain tumor biopsy, deep brain stimulation for Parkinson's disease, and psychological treatment.

Yashoda Hospitals, Hyderabad

One of Hyderabad's top multi-specialty hospitals is Yashoda Hospitals.   Yashoda Group of Hospitals has been offering high-quality healthcare for the people's various medical requirements over the past three decades. They have three branches in the city and its suburbs where they assist the residents of Hyderabad. Clinical quality, the best doctors and surgeons, and constantly improving, trying to cut facilities and services are the strengths of this facility. Modern facilities and latest technology provide 3600 patients with the greatest care and outcomes in healthcare. The best resources are available at Yashoda Neuro Institute for treating patients with serious nervous system injuries(*Best Hospitals in Hyderabad, India | Yashoda Hospitals, Somajiguda,* n.d.).

They are speciality in

Epilepsy

Cerebrovascular Disorders

Movement Disorder

Dementia

Stroke

Neuroimmunology

Traumatic Brain Injury

Brain Tumors, etc.

Awards and Recognitions:
NABH accredited hospital

NABL certificated labs

Won the No.1 Best Multi-specialty Hospital in the first edition of the Times Healthcare Achievers Telugu States award in 2017

Hospital was awarded with 1st Best Multispecialty hospital in Hyderabad, India in The Week Nielsen Best Hospital Survey for 2015

Apollo Health City, Jubilee Hills

Apollo Healthcare, which was founded by Dr. Prathap C. Reddy in 1983, is well-known in the healthcare field. With the best clinical outcomes, Apollo Hospitals has touched more than 120 million people from over 120 countries, providing everything from everyday wellness and preventative health care to innovative life-saving treatments and diagnostic services.

The neurology department of Apollo Health City is the most efficient and well-equipped to handle any neurological problems. The best place for neurology and neurosurgery in Hyderabad is due to their experience, number, success rates, and number of surgeries performed. The department of neurology includes specialized imaging, electrophysiological, and lab resources for diagnostic. Apollo Hospital Center, a dedicated neurology and neurosurgery hospital in Hyderabad, provides successful treatments for a variety of problems, including migraine, multiple sclerosis, multiple vascular disease, epilepsy, movement disorders, and neuromuscular diseases.

Specialties:

Children's Neurology

Epilepsy

Cardiology Neuro

Stereotactic Radiosurgery

Stroke Treatment

Neuropsychology

back ache that is neuropathic

Parkinson's disease

Dementia

Dystonia

Continental Hospital, Gachibowli

JCI and NABH recognized Continental Hospital provides multispecialty, tertiary, and quaternary care services. Dr. Guru N. Reddy started Continental Hospitals in April 2013 with the aim of changing healthcare in India by offering high-quality patient care with honesty, openness, a team-based approach, and evidence-based medicine. Gastroenterology, oncology, orthopedics, neuroscience, cardiology, and multi-organ transplants are major specialities. The best neurological hospital in Hyderabad for the treatment of neurological problems is Continental Hospitals.

Excellent neurosurgeons that specialize in brain, nerve, or spinal cord surgery are also available at Continental Hospitals. They have the most advanced operating microscope and neuronavigation, which help neurosurgeons in locating damaged brain regions and treating them without harming the important parts of the brain. Using sophisticated Neurophysiology (EMG, NCV, EEG) technology and video-EEG diagnostic methods(*Continental Hospitals | Multispeciality Hospital in Hyderabad | Best Hospital in Hyderabad | Best Multispeciality Hospital Gachibowli Hyderabad India*, n.d.).

The hospital won both the "National Excellence in Healthcare Award" and "The Best Multi Specialty Hospital of the Year" awards on March 31, 2014, at the Indo-Global Healthcare Summit.

On January 19, 2014, in Delhi, it also won the "Green Hospital of the Year" Award at the India Green Business Summit & Awards.

Specialties:

Continental Emergency Stroke Program

 Micro-neurosurgery

Brain Tumors

Head and Neck Surgeries

Vascular Surgery

Traumatic Brain Injuries

Minimally Invasive Surgeries

Stereotactic Surgery

Movement Disorders

Intensive Trauma Management

Spinal Surgeries

leep Disorders

Prathima Hospital

Since 15 years, Prathima Hospitals have been ranked as the best hospital in Hyderabad. PRATIMA has a long history of providing outstanding medical education and healthcare services. The Neurology & Neurosurgery Department at PRATHIMA is properly equipped to handle problems affecting the brain, spinal cord, muscles, and nerves. also provide high surgical and non-invasive treatments(Multispeciality Hospital in Hyderabad | About Us | Prathima Hospitals, n.d.). For the diagnosis and treatment of different neurological disorders, highest outpatient and inpatient services are offered. Epilepsy, neuromuscular diseases, pediatric stroke, neonatal neurology, developmental disorders, Parkinson's disease, Alzheimer's disease, stroke, dementia, multiple sclerosis, Parkinson's disease, Parkinson's disease, neuromuscular diseases, and spine disorders are just a few of the neurological conditions that a skilled team of doctors in our hospital treat. Various researches are offered by the neurophysiology department, including electrophysiological tests, EEG, nerve conduction tests, CT scans, and MRI scans. CT scans and MRI scans are available approximately, and the OT is equipped with a C-arm, a high-speed drill, and micro-instruments.

Nikhil Hospital

For providing patients with best neurology services over the past ten years, Nikhil Hospital has become one of Hyderabad's Best Neurology Hospitals. Dr. Nikhil Sunkarineni, one of the best neurologists in Hyderabad, is in head of the team of neurologists, who are some of the brightest in the field. Known for providing the best neurology care, Nikhil Neurology Hospital is a tertiary care hospital with the goal of providing patients with the highest level of consideration, care, and dedication.(*Best Neurology Hospital in Hyderabad | Nikhil Hospitals*, n.d.)

Siddarth Neuro Center

A neurology hospital called Siddarth Neuro Center is located in Chanda Nagar, Hyderabad.

The Siddarth Neuro Hospital is a complete facility that combines medical technology with a committed staff of healthcare experts to treat disorders of the spine and brain. Highly skilled neurologists, neurosurgeons, neurointerventionists, neuro-anesthetists, neurocritical care specialists, neuropsychologists, and neuropsychiatrists are on work at the institute. The Siddarth Neuro Hospital features specialized centers for headache, stroke, epilepsy, mobility problems, and brain tumors. For the emergency treatment of acute neurological disorders, such as stroke and other neurological injuries, the institute has specific services and procedures. Sidarth Hospitals' Department of Neurology provides patients of all ages with quality healthcare for conditions that affect the brain, spinal cord, muscles, and nerves. The article efficiently addresses a wide range of nervous system ailments, including dementia, Parkinson's disease, sleep disorders, neuropathies, headache, stroke, epilepsy, vertigo, neck and back pain, and other chronic aches. It also discusses many other neuromuscular disorders. Moreover, it treats neurological issues in children such cerebral palsy, delayed development, mental retardation, and behavior problems(*Best Neurology Hospital In Hyderabad | Sidarth Hospitals*, n.d.).

As a committed neurology and neurosurgery facility in Hyderabad, Sidarth Hospitals provides efficient treatments and initiatives for conditions such as epilepsy, Parkinson's disease, neuromuscular diseases, brain tumors, spine disorders, multiple sclerosis, headaches, migraine headaches, and others that affect the nervous system.

Neehar Epilepsy Center

The neurology-specific hospital in KPHB, Hyderabad, is called Neehar Neuro. Injuries like headaches, neck pain, back pain, epilepsy, unconscious spells, muscle weakness, tingling and paraesthesia, numbness, thinning of a part of the body, sleeplessness, memory loss, vertigo/spinning sensation, posture or walking difficulties (Parkinson's disease or balance disorders), tremors, speech difficulty, and developmental problems are some of the conditions researchers analyze and manage treatment for it. The Neuro Center focuses in the identification and management of diseases that affect the brain, spinal cord, muscles, and nerves. As the top neurologist in Hyderabad, they have grown in status because to the dedication to giving patients the finest quality of care.

Hyderabad MultiSpeciality Hospital (HMH)

The Hyderabad MultiSpeciality Hospital in Malakpet is famous hospital in the area; rather, it represents an effort to increase and expand the devotion and dedication of Dr. A. Vishnu Vardhan Reddy, who has been giving his patients quality care in the field of urology for the past 20 years. HMH Neurosciences is a complete treatment and research facility for all types of neurological diseases. They treat problems of the spinal cord, brain, and peripheral nerves. Their neurological department, a center of medical innovation, is equipped with the most advanced neuro-imaging and diagnostic technology. specialized care for patients with a variety of neurologic disorders, including amyotrophic lateral sclerosis, epilepsy, Parkinson's disease, Parkinson's disease-related dementias, Parkinson's disease, and other movement disorders. Current neuro-intensive care facilities and neuroradiology services help neurologists and neurosurgeons reach neurological disease & treatment outcomes that are equivalent to those of the best institutions in the world(*Hyderabad MultiSpeciality Hospital | Best Orthopedic Hospitals in Hyderabad*, n.d.).

At HMH, Our neurosurgery doctors treat diseases such as

Brain injury or diseases

Head injury

Brain hemorrhage

Tumors

Disc prolapse or herniation

Spinal tumors

Spinal dislocation

Spinal injury

Unstable spine

Brain tumors

Nerve injuries

Hydrocephalus

HMH utilizes the most up-to-date infrastructure and equipment for invasive, noninvasive, and critical care, rehabilitation, and general patient care. neuro-intensive care services include:

Ventilators

5 Tesla MRI

ICP monitors

Electroencephalography (EEG)

Neuro-Diagnostics

Online monitors

Carotid Doppler

Central oxygen & suction

Dual Source CT Scan

Digital Subtraction Angiography (DSA)

Over the years, a number of new methods have been developed to cure diseases that were considered incurable and to improve the safety of neurological treatments.

CHAPTER 6: DRUG MANUFACTRING INDUSTRIES IN TELANGANA

India is currently the second-largest provider of employees for the global biotech and pharmaceutical sectors. The Indian pharmaceutical industry supplies more than half of the world's demand for various vaccinations, as well as 25% of the UK's total pharmaceutical market and 40% of the US market for generic drugs. In the world, India exports 20% of all generic medications. India's pharmaceutical business includes biopharmaceuticals, bioservices, bioagriculture, bio industry, and bioinformatics.(*Pharma – Invest Telangana*, n.d.).

In India, Telangana is the centre for pharmaceutical manufacturing industry since it has 35 to 40% of the total population of India. This got only improved after Hyderabad Pharma city is established. Major pharmaceutical companies like Mylan NV, Albany Molecular Research Inc., and Cambrex Corp has their production sites in Telangana. Hyderabad is also known has a life science capital of India. In life science industry Telangana has received more than Rs 10,000 crore in investment. Telangana's pharmaceutical and biotechnology sector is expected to reach 9 lakh crores.(*Andhra Pradesh and Telangana Are Manufacturing Powerhouses for US API Supply*, n.d.)

According to Telangana minister KT Rama Rao for IT and industries, Telangana is a state with a strong economy which is suitable to fast industry expansion, also a strong pharmaceutical industry. Hyderabad is also known as the "Vaccine Capital of the Globe". And also played a significant part in providing vaccinations during the pandemic. Also, the fact that the State contributes to more than 40% of pharmaceutical manufacturing.

There are more than 800 pharmaceutical companies in Telangana, and some of the top pharma industries are listed below.

Gland Pharma limited

Gland Pharma limited has established in 1978 in Hyderabad under the company act 1956. Over time, it has developed from a contract manufacturer of low volume liquid parenteral pharmaceuticals to one of the biggest and most expanding rapidly manufactures of prescription injectables. The company's main business is the production of injectable formulations. The company operates seven manufacturing facilities in India, including three API facilities, four finished formulations facilities, and four facilities with a combined 22 production lines. The company had a manufacturing capacity for finished formulations of about 755 million units annually as of March 31 2020. (*Global Injectable Manufacturer & Supplier | CDMO Pharma Company | Gland Pharma Limited*, n.d.)As a fully integrated business, the company has strong production skills as well as internal research and development (R&D) experience. a strict quality control process, significant regulatory knowledge, and established marketing and distribution connections. They specialize in complex injectables such as NCE-1s, First-to-File products, and 505(b)(2) filings and are present in the sterile injectables, oncology, and ophthalmic segments.

SMS Pharmaceuticals Ltd.

a global integrated pharmaceutical organization with operations in over 70 nations. With a strong research and production staff and state-of-the-art facilities, SMS

Pharmaceuticals Ltd. is a major participant in the world of API manufacture. SMS is dedicated to provide its customers with the best value possible in the most efficient manner. In order to meet its organization style and fulfill USFDA and WHO cGMP requirements, the company over time created incredible manufacturing facilities. There are currently four facilities running. They can work with a wide variety of APIs and intermediates, and they have experience working with a variety of process reactions and reactor volumes up to 15 KL(*API – SMS Pharmaceuticals Ltd*, n.d.). At each manufacturing facility, SMS has established fully working quality control cells staffed by knowledgeable and experienced personnel. Wet labs, instrumentation labs, and microbiology labs are available in each of these QA/QC blocks to conduct intermediate, in-process, and final product analyses. A global pharmaceutical corporation with operations in over 70 nations, SMS Pharmaceuticals is integrated.

Aurobindo Pharma

Aurobindo Pharma was established in 1986 as a result of a vision shared by Mr. P. V. Ramprasad Reddy, Mr. K. Nityananda Reddy, and a small group of extremely dedicated experts.

It was initially approved in China by our plant in India.

Also Phase III PCV clinical studies were started. And purchased nine OTC brands. its first biosimilar application was submitted to the European Medical Agency (EMA). The company makes both active medicinal components and generic medications. Aurobindo Pharma is also active in several important therapeutic areas, including gastrointestinal, cephalosporins, anti-retrovirals, cardiology, and neurosciences. On October 7, 2019, Aurobindo said that the USFDA has issued seven observations for its unit-7 formulation factory in Telangana for potentially inaccurate paperwork.

Sri Krishna Pharmaceuticals Ltd (SKPL)

Sri Krishna Pharmaceuticals Ltd (SKPL), established in 1974 by Dr.V.V. Subba Reddy to manufacture Paracetmol. Acetaminophen (Paracetamol) is manufactured in large quantities for the Indian domestic market. In 1985 it also expanded by manufacturing folic acid(*Sri Krishna Pharmaceuticals Limited - Manufacturer from Uppal, Hyderabad, India | About Us*, n.d.).Additionally, it specializes in producing first line defense Active Pharmaceutical

Ingredients(APIs) to PFIs and finished dosage drugs in bulk. The company is still the largest manufacturer of the paracetamol and company has 201-500 employee. Its special services asre API and FDF.

Manufacturing facilities like Acetaminophen/ Paracetamol (APAP) is carried out by Dedicated facilities without exposure to an uncontrolled environment outside, with closed vacuum transfer systems and forced ventilation systems. so it is approved by the TGA, Australia.

Some of their products are: Paracetamol, Aspirin, , Follic Acid, Ibuprofen, Glyburide, Naproxen, Furosemide, , Metformin, Glipizide and Meclizine Hydrochlroide etc.

Rakshit Private Limited

Rakshit Private Limited is estasblished in the year 2000 with strong manufacturer of an integrated APIs and it is intermediates for global market. It is one of the leading company in Telangana. distributing its goods globally from the United States to Europe, Japan, Asia, and Latin America. Rakshit has also submitted Certificate of Suitability(CEP) for its main products. As the biggest producer of sildenafil citrate, it has made a name for itself and aims to lead the industry in all the products it produces.Additionally, reputable organizations including CDSCO India, Japan PMDA, Korea MFDS, and USFDA have approved its facilities. Rakshit is dedicated to maintaining the highest standard of quality in the development and production of pharmaceutical goods(*Rakshit Drugs - Pharmaceutical Company in Hyderabad*, n.d.).

Biological E Ltd

It is founded by Dr. DVK Raju in 1953 and it is the top company in Telangana. It is manufacturing products like live extracts and anti coagulants. In 1962 it is the first Indian company to start vaccine business . it has also manufacturing for liquid orals, solid dosage forms and syrups, API, and parental(*Biological E Ltd*, n.d.)

LEE Pharma Ltd

It is established in the year 1997 on 6th October in Hyderabad with share capital is Rs. 76, 500,000. It has larged its position in the global market and phenomenal growth rate with the product innovation and dedicated teams. They produce Active Pharmaceutical Ingredients (API), capsules, ointments, granules , pellets and finished formulations(*LEE PHARMA*

*LIMITED - Company, Directors and Contact Details |
Zauba Corp*, n.d.)

HI-Tech pharmaceuticals

It was established in the year 1985 in Hyderabad with share capital INR 45,000,000. Ii has mainly focused on three areas that are nutrition, poultry animals, health management for aquatic.   Their main products are Azithromycin, Deflazacort(*Deflazacort Drug Information - Indications, Dosage, Side Effects and Precautions*, n.d.).

Mars therapeutic and chemicals ltd

Mars Therapeutics Private Limited is a Pharmaceutical Company established in Hyderabad, India in 1993. With thirty years of experience in the manufacturing and marketing of pharmaceuticals. It manufactures are primarily into oral finished dosages (Tablets, Capsules, and Liquids) and semi-finished dosages (DC Granules). It exports finished dosages and Granules to countries in Europe, South East Asia, Middle East, CIS, Africa, Latin America(*Mars Therapeutics Private Limited*, n.d.).

Accrete Pharmaceuticals Private Limited

Accrete Pharmaceuticals Private Limited was established in Hyderabad, India in 2005. Aita Srinivas is the founder of Accrete Pharmaceuticals Private Limited. Their main focuses were on anti- cancer products. It is majorly in Manufacturing (Metals & Chemicals, and products thereof) business(*Accrete Pharmaceuticals Private Limited*, n.d.).

MSN laboratories pvt ltd

MSN Group is the research-based pharmaceutical company based out of India established in 2003. Their vision is to constantly delivering affordable world class medicines. Dr MSN Reddy is the managing director of MSN groups. They have achieved 300+ Formulations, covering over 35 major therapies(*Who We Are - MSN Laboratories | Leading Pharmaceutical Company*, n.d.).

Hetero drugs ltd

Hetero drugs started in 1993 as an API player in the Indian Pharmaceutical market. Founded by Dr BPS Reddy in Hyderabad. They are now largest producers of APIs globally and a leader in ARV APIs and FDFs. It has a wide range of products in therapeutic categories including HIV/AIDS, Oncology, Cardiovascular, Hepatitis, Neurology, Biosimilars, COVID-19, Immunology, Gastroenterology, Urology, Respiratory, Diabetes, Allergy, Malaria, Ophthalmology, Haematology, Autoimmune Disorders(*Hetero Drugs Ltd. | Devex*, n.d.).

Biophore

Biophore was established in 29 March 2007. (Biophore) was founded by Dr Jagadeesh Babu and Dr Manik Reddy. Their aim is to place Biophore in the most reliable knowledge-based firms in the API sector. Their Products are Oncology, Contrast agents, Peptides, Injectable APIs, Orphan Drugs(*Biophore India Pharmaceuticals Overview and Company Profile | AmbitionBox*, n.d.).

Suven Pharmaceuticals Ltd

It is established on 6th nov 2018. It is a biopharmaceutical company. Its main research is on Central Nervous System(CNS) disorder and also manufacturing of New Chemical entity with Active Pharmaceutical Ingredient (API)(*Suven Pharmaceuticals Company History - Business Standard News | Page 1*, n.d.)

Eugia pharma specialists limited

It was established on 17th April 2013 based in Hyderabad. it has share capital of Rs. 8,000,000,000 and paid up capital is Rs. 6,210,086,900. Its primary areas of development are in cancer and hormonal generic formulation(*Eugia Pharma Specialities Limited - Company Details | The Company Check*, n.d.).

Laurus labs ltd

Laurus labs ltd was founded in 2005 by Dr.Satyanarayana Chava. The company headquarters is in Hyderabad. Its focus areas are active pharmaceutical ingredients (APIs), generic formulations, custom synthesis and biotechnology. The company also makes Dolutegravir/lamivudine/tenofovir, a medication for HIV/AIDS, and hydroxychloroquine tablets, which are used to treat certain types of malaria(*ABOUT US | Laurus Labs*, n.d.).

Granules India ltd

Granules India ltd was formed in 1984 as Triton Laboratories. Mr Krishna prasad Chigurupati is the founder of Granules. Its headquarters is in Hyderabad It manufactures several off-patent drugs, including Paracetamol, Ibuprofen, Metformin and Guaifenesin, on a large scale for customers(*Granulesindia*, n.d.).

Qualitek pharma

Qualitek pharma was established in 2005. They are well known in producing best quality Sustained and Modified Release Pellets, Taste Masked Granules(*Qualitek Pharma*, n.d.).

Natco pharma ltd

Natco pharma ltd was established in 1981. VC Nannapaneni is the founder of Natco Pharma. The company manufactures finished dosage formulations activepharmaceutical ingredients (API) and crop health science products.It is a major producer of branded oncology medicines and hepatitis C drugs. (*Natco Pharma* |, n.d.).

Therdose pharma pvt ltd

Therdose pharma pvt ltd was founded in 2003. Dr. Nagesh Palepu is the founder of Therdose Pharma.

TherDose is a generic cancer drugs developer, manufacturer, marketer, and exporter with strong in-house expertise and state-of-the-art R&D facilities(*Therdose Pharma Private Limited - Company Details | The Company Check*, n.d.).

Neuland laboratories ltd

Neuland laboratories ltd was established in 1984. Davuluri Rama Mohan Rao was the founder of Neuland. Their mainly Focusing on API capabilities and providing services such as cost-effective synthesis, IP protection(*Neuland Labs*, n.d.).

Alembic global research pvt ltd

Alembic global research pvt ltd was founded in 1907. The company has its headquarters and office situated in Vadodara, Gujarat, India. It is also termed to be a market leader in macrolides segment of anti-infective drugs in India(*Alembic Pharmaceutical | Pharmaceutical Company*, n.d.).

Optimus generic ltd

Optimus generic ltd was established in 2004. Dr. D. Srinivas Reddy was the founder of Optimus generic. Optimus is an integrated manufacturer of pharmaceutical products including advanced intermediates, APIs and finished drug.

Aurore life science pvt ltd

Aurore life science pvt ltd was established in 2010. Headquarters located in Hyderabad. It focuses on the area of Active pharmaceutical Ingredient (API). The USFDA approved the first Indian company in 1994 to make OTC and prescription drugs for the US market.

Smilax laboratories ltd

It is established in the year 2004. The company is selling antidepressants, psychostimulants, ulcer-causing, fungal, migraine, platelet, anginal, and pellet drugs(Maciej Serda et al., 2013)

Ammana bio pharma ltd

Ammana bio pharma ltd was established in Oct 1994.it manufactures ethanol products for the oil industry(*Ammana Bio Pharma Ltd - Company Profile and News - Bloomberg Markets*, n.d.).

Emmennar pharma pvt ltd

Emmennar pharma pvt ltd was established in 2005. Ravi Dutt Sharma is the Managing director of Emmennar. It is the Manufacturer of Fiber drums which used to pack the API's.

Both Indian and international major companies have chosen Telangana as their preferred location for investments in the pharma industry.

REFERENCES

ABOUT US | Laurus Labs. (n.d.). Retrieved September 21, 2022, from https://www.lauruslabs.com/about

Accrete Pharmaceuticals Private Limited. (n.d.). Retrieved September 21, 2022, from https://www.accretepharma.com/about-us.html

Aim & Scope - (IAIM). (n.d.). Retrieved September 16, 2022, from https://www.iaimjournal.com/

Alembic Pharmaceutical | Pharmaceutical Company. (n.d.). Retrieved September 21, 2022, from https://alembicpharmaceuticals.com/

Ammana Bio Pharma Ltd - Company Profile and News - Bloomberg Markets. (n.d.). Retrieved September 19, 2022, from https://www.bloomberg.com/profile/company/ABPL:IN

Andhra Pradesh and Telangana are manufacturing powerhouses for US API supply. (n.d.). Retrieved September 17, 2022, from https://www.globaldata.com/andhra-pradesh-and-telangana-are-manufacturing-powerhouses-for-us-api-supply/

API – SMS Pharmaceuticals Ltd. (n.d.). Retrieved September 17, 2022, from https://smspharma.com/api/

Best Hospital For Epilepsy Treatment Surgery in Hyderabad. (n.d.). Retrieved September 17, 2022, from https://www.kimshospitals.com/secunderabad/speciality/epilepsy-centre/

Best Hospitals in Hyderabad, India | Yashoda Hospitals, Somajiguda. (n.d.). Retrieved September 17, 2022, from https://www.yashodahospitals.com/location/somajiguda/

Best Neurology Hospital in Hyderabad | Nikhil Hospitals. (n.d.). Retrieved September 17, 2022, from https://www.nikhilhospitals.com/

Best Neurology Hospital In Hyderabad | Sidarth Hospitals. (n.d.). Retrieved September 17, 2022, from *Best Neurology Hospital in Hyderabad | Top Neurology in Hyderabad*. (n.d.). Retrieved September 16, 2022, from https://www.kimshospitals.com/secunderabad/speciality/neurology/

Best Pediatric Neurologist in Hyderabad | Dr Habib Pathan |. (n.d.). Retrieved September 16, 2022, from https://www.drhabibpediatricneurologist.com/

Biological E Ltd. (n.d.). Retrieved September 18, 2022, from https://www.biologicale.com/

Biophore India Pharmaceuticals Overview and Company Profile | AmbitionBox. (n.d.). Retrieved September 21, 2022, from https://www.ambitionbox.com/overview/biophore-india-pharmaceuticals-overview

Buckley, A. W., & Holmes, G. L. (2016). Epilepsy and autism. *Cold Spring Harbor Perspectives in Medicine,* *6*(4). https://doi.org/10.1101/CSHPERSPECT.A022749

Burden of neurological disorders have doubled in 30 years in India. (n.d.). Retrieved September 15, 2022, from https://www.deccanchronicle.com/science/scienc

e/150721/burden-of-neurological-disorders-have-doubled-in-30-years-in-india.html

Continental Hospitals | Multispeciality Hospital in Hyderabad | Best Hospital in Hyderabad | Best Multispeciality Hospital Gachibowli Hyderabad India. (n.d.). Retrieved September 17, 2022, from https://continentalhospitals.com/

Deflazacort Drug Information - Indications, Dosage, Side Effects and Precautions. (n.d.). Retrieved September 18, 2022, from https://www.medindia.net/doctors/drug_information/deflazacort.htm

Dr. K. Krishna Reddy - Neurosurgeon in Hyderabad | ClinicSpots. (n.d.). Retrieved September 16, 2022, from https://www.clinicspots.com/doctor/dr-k-reddy-14

Dr. M.Chandra Sekhar Reddy, Neurologist - Kukatpally, Hyderabad. | Drlogy. (n.d.). Retrieved September 16, 2022, from https://drlogy.com/doctors/dr-m.chandra-sekhar-reddy-24224

Dr. Neehar Potluri - Neurologist - Book Appointment

Online, View Fees, Feedbacks | Practo. (n.d.). Retrieved September 16, 2022, from https://www.practo.com/hyderabad/doctor/dr-neehar-potluri-neurologist?practice_id=654998&specialization=Epilepsy&referrer=doctor_listing&category_name=symptom&category_id=41

Dr. R. N. Komal Kumar,Neurologist in Secunderabad,Hyderabad Reviews,Contact Number,Fees | 365Doctor. (n.d.). Retrieved September 16, 2022, from https://www.365doctor.in/doctor/dr-r-n-komal-kumar-neurologist

Dr. Sandhya Manorenj - Neurologist - Book Appointment Online, View Fees, Feedbacks | Practo. (n.d.). Retrieved September 16, 2022, from https://www.practo.com/hyderabad/doctor/sandhya-manorenj

Dr. Subhash Kaul | Best Neuro Surgeon in Hyderabad | Alzheimers Specialist in Hyderabad. (n.d.). Retrieved September 21, 2022, from https://www.kimshospitals.com/doctor-profile/dr-subhash-kaul/

Dr. Sujit Kumar Vidiyala - Neurosurgeon - Book Appointment Online, View Fees, Feedbacks | Practo. (n.d.). Retrieved September 16, 2022, from https://www.practo.com/hyderabad/doctor/dr-sujit-kumar-vidiyala-neurosurgeon

Dr. Suma K. - Neurologist - Book Appointment Online, View Fees, Feedbacks | Practo. (n.d.). Retrieved September 16, 2022, from https://www.practo.com/hyderabad/doctor/dr-kandukuri-suma

Dr. Suresh Babu Consultant Neurologist & Epileptologist in Hyderabad. (n.d.). Retrieved September 21, 2022, from https://aighospitals.com/doctors/dr-suresh-babu/

Dr Amitava Ray | Neurosurgeon in Hyderabad - Apollo Health City Jubilee Hills. (n.d.). Retrieved September 21, 2022, from https://www.askapollo.com/doctors/neurosurgeon/hyderabad/dr-amitava-ray

Dr Pranathi Gutta | Paediatric Neurologist in

Hyderabad - Apollo Health City Jubilee Hills. (n.d.). Retrieved September 21, 2022, from https://www.askapollo.com/doctors/paediatric-neurologist/hyderabad/dr-pranathi-gutta

Eugia Pharma Specialities Limited - Company Details | The Company Check. (n.d.). Retrieved September 18, 2022, from https://www.thecompanycheck.com/company/eugia-pharma-specialities-limited/U24297TG2013PLC087048

Experts say Telangana needs more neurologists- The New Indian Express. (n.d.). Retrieved September 16, 2022, from https://www.newindianexpress.com/states/telangana/2022/jul/22/experts-say-telangana-needs-more-neurologists-2479320.html

Global Injectable Manufacturer & Supplier | CDMO Pharma Company | Gland Pharma Limited. (n.d.). Retrieved September 17, 2022, from https://glandpharma.com/

Gourie-Devi, M. (2014). Epidemiology of neurological disorders in India: Review of background, prevalence and incidence of epilepsy, stroke, *Parkinson's disease* and tremors. *Neurology India,* 62(6), 588. https://doi.org/10.4103/0028-3886.149365

GSDP: Telangana's GSDP more than doubles to Rs 11.55 lakh cr in 8 yrs - The Economic Times. (n.d.).

Hetero Drugs Ltd. | Devex. (n.d.). Retrieved September 21, 2022, from https://www.devex.com/organizations/hetero-drugs-ltd-45606

Huge challenges ahead for new Telangana tourism corporation | Hyderabad News - Times of India. (n.d.).

Hyderabad MultiSpeciality Hospital | Best Orthopedic Hospitals in Hyderabad. (n.d.). Retrieved September 17, 2022, from https://www.hmhcare.com/

Journal, I. (n.d.). *A Study on Clinical Profile of New Onset Focal Seizures in a Tertiary Care Centre.* Retrieved September 16, 2022, from https://www.academia.edu/15024769/A_Study_o n_Clinical_Profile_of_New_Onset_Focal_Seizure s_in_a_Tertiary_Care_Centre

Kims Hospitals. (n.d.-a). Retrieved September 17, 2022, from https://www.kimshospitals.com/secunderabad/speciality/epilepsy-centre/technology/

Kims Hospitals. (n.d.-b). Retrieved September 17, 2022, from https://www.kimshospitals.com/blog/refractory-epilepsy/

LEE PHARMA LIMITED - Company, directors and contact details | Zauba Corp. (n.d.). Retrieved September 18, 2022, from https://www.zaubacorp.com/company/LEE-PHARMA-LIMITED/U24230TG1997PLC028095

Mars Therapeutics Private Limited. (n.d.). Retrieved September 21, 2022, from http://marspharma.co.in/about-us.php

Multispeciality Hospital in Hyderabad | About Us | Prathima Hospitals. (n.d.). Retrieved September 17, 2022, from https://prathimahospitals.com/best-hospital-in-hyderabad/

Natco Pharma |. (n.d.). Retrieved September 21, 2022, from https://www.natcopharma.co.in/

Neuro Specialist Hyderabad | Best Neurologist In Hyderabad. (n.d.). Retrieved September 16, 2022, from https://www.kimshospitals.com/doctor-profile/dr-sita-jayalakshmi/

Pappala, B. C. S., Indugula, J. P., Talabhatula, S. K., Kolli, R. S., Shrivastava, A. K., & Sahu, P. S. (2016). Diagnosis of neurocysticercosis among patients with seizures in northern coastal districts of Andhra Pradesh, India. *Asian Pacific Journal of Tropical Biomedicine,* 6(11), 903–908. https://doi.org/10.1016/J.APJTB.2016.09.001

Pharma – Invest Telangana. (n.d.). Retrieved September 17, 2022, from https://invest.telangana.gov.in/pharma/

Qualitek Pharma. (n.d.). Retrieved September 21, 2022, from https://www.qualitekpharma.com/

Rakshit Drugs - Pharmaceutical Company in Hyderabad. (n.d.). Retrieved September 21, 2022, from https://rakshitdrugspvtltd.com/

Sastry, C. P. V. R., & Reddy, R. M. (2018). Study of prevalence and clinical spectrum of seizures in children in a teaching hospital in rural Telangana, India. *International Journal of Contemporary Pediatrics*, 5(3), 862–866. https://doi.org/10.18203/2349-3291.ijcp20181503

Seshan, K. S. S. (2018). Telangana: History and the formation of a new state. *Https://Doi.Org/10.1177/2348448918759870*, 5(1), 72–82. https://doi.org/10.1177/2348448918759870

'Shortage of neurologists in country' - The Hindu. (n.d.). Retrieved September 16, 2022, from https://www.thehindu.com/news/national/telangana/shortage-of-neurologists-in-country/article29588579.ece

Sri Krishna Pharmaceuticals Limited - Manufacturer from Uppal, Hyderabad, India | About Us. (n.d.). Retrieved September 18, 2022, from https://www.indiamart.com/sri-krishna-pharmaceuticals/aboutus.html

Stafstrom, C. E., & Carmant, L. (2015). Seizures and

Epilepsy: An Overview for Neuroscientists. *Cold Spring Harbor Perspectives in Medicine*, 5(6), 1–19. https://doi.org/10.1101/CSHPERSPECT.A022426

Suven Pharmaceuticals Company History - Business Standard News | Page 1. (n.d.). Retrieved September 18, 2022, from https://www.business-standard.com/company/suven-pharma-74679/information/company-history

Telangana | encyclopedia article by TheFreeDictionary. (n.d.).

Telangana | History, Map, Population, Capital, & Government | Britannica. (n.d.).

Telangana among Top-10 global startup ecosystems. (n.d.).

Telangana State Portal History. (n.d.).

Telangana to spend Rs 10,000 crore on improving public healthcare | Deccan Herald. (n.d.). Retrieved September 19, 2022, from https://www.deccanherald.com/national/south/tel

angana-to-spend-rs-10000-crore-on-improving-public-healthcare-1050263.html

The Telangana People's Movement: The Unfolding Political Culture on JSTOR. (n.d.). Retrieved September 20, 2022, from https://www.jstor.org/stable/20787475

Therdose Pharma Private Limited - Company Details | The Company Check. (n.d.). Retrieved September 21, 2022, from https://www.thecompanycheck.com/company/therdose-pharma-private-limited/U24239TG2003PTC042272

9 798355 336493